SCIENCE ON THE EDGE

FORENSICS

WRITTEN BY
JOANNE MATTERN

BLACKBIRCH®
PRESS

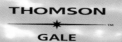

San Diego • Detroit • New York • San Francisco • Cleveland • New Haven, Conn. • Waterville, Maine • London • Munich

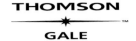

For more information, contact
The Gale Group, Inc.
27500 Drake Rd.
Farmington Hills, MI 48331-3535
Or you can visit our Internet site at http://www.gale.com

Photo credits: cover © Getty Images; pages 7, 8-9, 12, 14, 17, 18, 24, 25, 27, 34, 36, 37, 38, 42, 43 © CORBIS; pages 5, 6, 11, 19, 21, 22, 23, 26, 28, 29, 30, 31, 32, 33, 35 © Mikael Karlsson, www.arresting images.com

LIBRARY OF CONGRESS CATALOGING-IN-PUBLICATION DATA

Mattern, Joanne, 1963-
   Forensics / by Joanne Mattern.
      p. cm. — (Science on the edge)
   Summary: Discusses the investigation by scientists and detectives of deaths that occur under mysterious circumstances, including how forensic science developed and how technology is transforming the field.
   Includes bibliographical references and index.
   ISBN 1-56711-785-6 (hardback : alk. paper)
   1. Forensic sciences—Juvenile literature. [1. Forensic sciences. 2. Criminal investigation.]
I. Title. II. Series: Science on the edge series.

   HV8073.M273 2004
   363.25—dc22   2003012995

Printed in United States
10 9 8 7 6 5 4 3 2 1

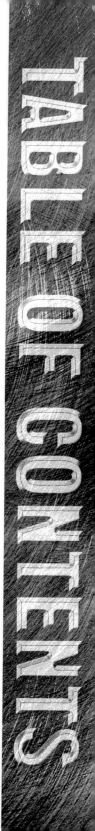

INTRODUCTION

FORENSIC SCIENCE

When a person dies under mysterious or suspicious circumstances, the death becomes a puzzle. Family and friends of the deceased, as well as the police, will wonder if the person died of natural causes or an accident, or if he or she was a victim of murder or suicide.

Some deaths raise even more questions. Sometimes when a body is discovered, the identity of the person is unknown. Investigators must determine who the person was, where the person was from, and how he or she arrived at the scene. If it is suspected that someone is responsible for the death, investigators must find out who the culprit is and where he or she can be found. In such cases, a team of detectives and scientists must piece together the clues from the scene and the body itself to solve any crime that may have been committed.

Forensic science can help solve many of these puzzles. Forensics is the application of science to the law, which means the use of science to solve a murder case, determine the cause of a mysterious death, or answer other important legal questions. Forensic scientists use clues left on the body and at the scene to determine how and why a person died, who the person was, and if any other person was connected to the death.

Forensic science has changed dramatically through the years. As recently as two hundred years ago, investigators used little more than their five senses to find clues and solve crimes. Today, high-tech laboratories, computer programs, and scientific procedures examine evidence that is too tiny for the human eye to see. These procedures can solve crimes and identify victims in cases that would have been impossible to figure out in years gone by.

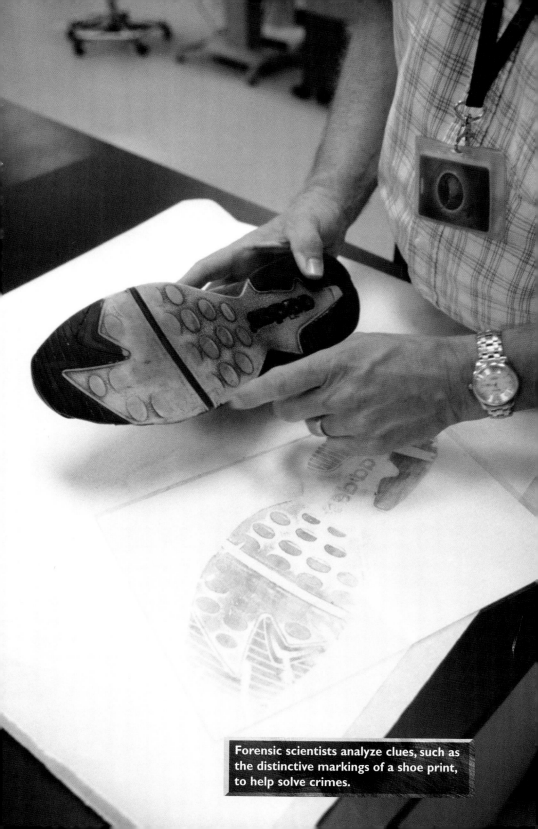

Forensic scientists analyze clues, such as the distinctive markings of a shoe print, to help solve crimes.

People have always been fascinated with the mysteries of life and death. The popularity of television shows such as *CSI* reveals how intriguing forensic science can be. This book takes a look at the history of forensic science—where it has been, where it is now, and where it is headed in the future.

High-tech equipment allows forensic scientists to examine evidence too small for the human eye to see.

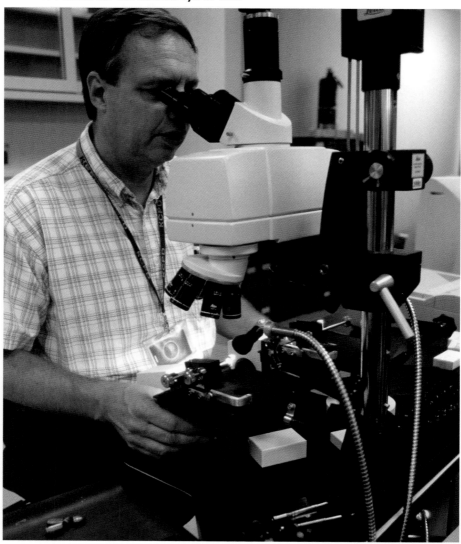

CHAPTER 1

FORENSICS THROUGH HISTORY
FORENSIC SCIENCE AND ITS CLUES

Forensic scientists uncover and use many different clues to solve their puzzles. At the scene of a death, they analyze the position of the body. Sometimes even the position of the furniture in the room can provide clues as to how the person died or if the body was brought to the scene from somewhere else. Nearby objects such as uneaten food or an empty bottle of medicine can be important clues to what the person was doing immediately prior to death.

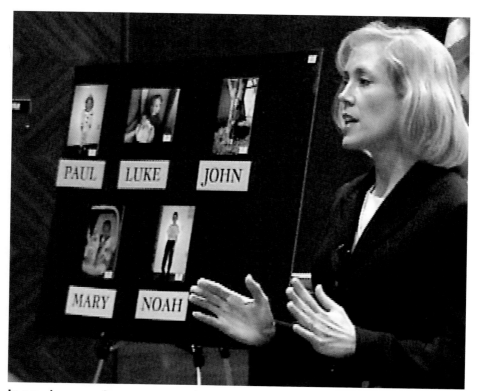

In murder cases, lawyers turn to forensic evidence to make connections between the crime and the accused person.

Forensic scientists also conduct a thorough examination of the body itself, which also holds clues that can explain how a person died. If it appears the person was murdered, forensic scientists look for evidence on the body left behind by the killer. Perhaps the victim scratched the killer and got some of the killer's skin under the fingernails; or perhaps the killer hit or bit the victim, and left telltale marks on the body.

The condition of the body also tells scientists when the person died and how long the body was left in the place in which it was found. Finally, fingerprints, dental work, scars, tattoos, and other details on the body can help identify the victim.

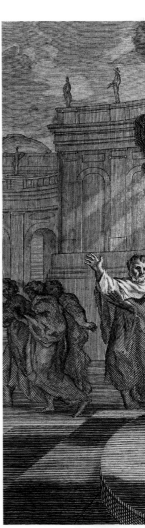

Once forensic scientists have gathered as many clues from the site and from the body as they can, they try to put the puzzle pieces together. Forensic scientists and detectives study all the evidence and then attempt to determine how and why the person died. If the death was a murder, forensic scientists might appear in court to explain what they found, why they think it points to a crime, and how the evidence connects the victim to the accused killer.

Forensic science is not new. In fact, people have used forensics to explain the causes and circumstances of death for thousands of years.

In 44 B.C., Antistius performed an autopsy of Julius Caesar's body, which revealed that only one of the emperor's twenty-three stab wounds was fatal.

EARLY FORENSICS TECHNIQUES

The first recorded autopsy was performed on Julius Caesar in 44 B.C. Caesar, the ruler of ancient Rome, was stabbed to death by several members of the Roman senate who wanted to seize power. Afterward, a doctor named Antistius studied the stab wounds and the damage they did to Caesar's body. Antistius concluded that although Caesar had been stabbed twenty-three times, only one wound, which went through the emperor's heart, was fatal.

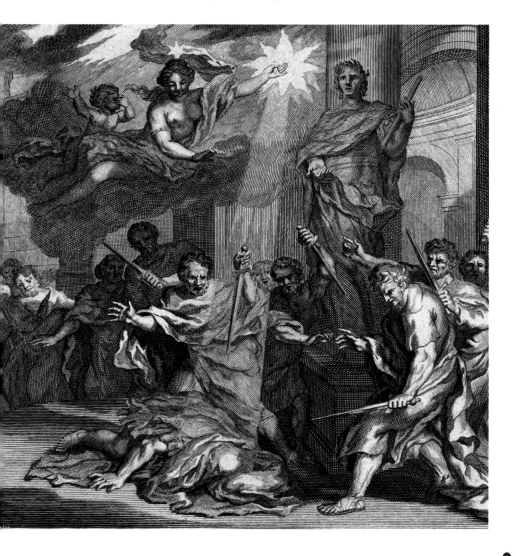

Although autopsies could determine the cause of death, they were not frequently performed in ancient times because many cultures believed that the body had to be in one piece for the person's soul to go to the afterlife. Because autopsies involve taking the body apart, they were viewed with horror and suspicion by many ancient cultures.

CORONERS AND THE FIRST FORENSICS TEXT

Despite the resistance to performing autopsies, people still wanted and needed to know what caused certain deaths. As a result, around A.D. 900, the position of coroner was developed in England. Originally, this position was called "keeper of the pleas of the crown" or "crowner" because the king could claim the property of a murderer or a suicide victim. The coroner's job was to decide whether a death was murder or suicide and inform the king.

In 1248, the first text about forensics, *The Washing Away of Wrongs*, was printed in China. It described ways to determine whether a death was natural or unnatural by observing details on the body. For example, it pointed out that a broken bone in the neck or marks on the throat could show that the victim had been strangled.

THE COMPOUND MICROSCOPE AND THE FIRST FORENSICS LAB

Scientists found a way to get a much closer look at the human body in 1590, when Zacharias Janssen invented the first compound microscope. Unlike a simple microscope with only one magnifying lens, the compound microscope used two or more lenses, which made it more powerful and enabled scientists to look at details that had been too tiny to see before.

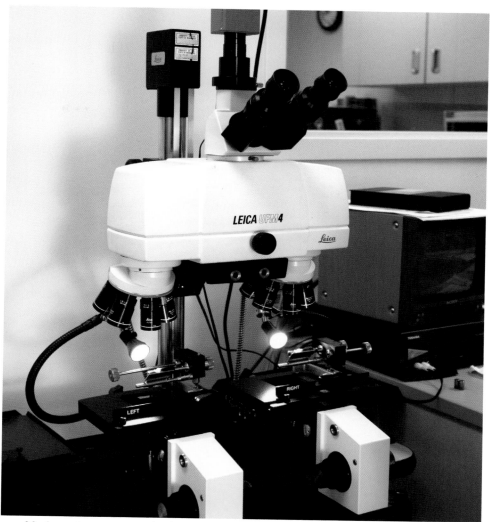

Modern-day compound microscopes, like the one pictured here, developed from Zacharias Janssen's 1590 invention that allowed scientists to see objects in greater detail.

In 1910, a Frenchman named Edmond Locard created the world's first forensics laboratory. Locard believed that a person who committed a crime always left something at the scene and always took something away. For example, a murder victim might have fibers of the killer's clothes on his or her body, or the killer might have bits of the victim's skin or blood under his or her fingernails. Locard's laboratory analyzed these small clues and used them to solve crimes.

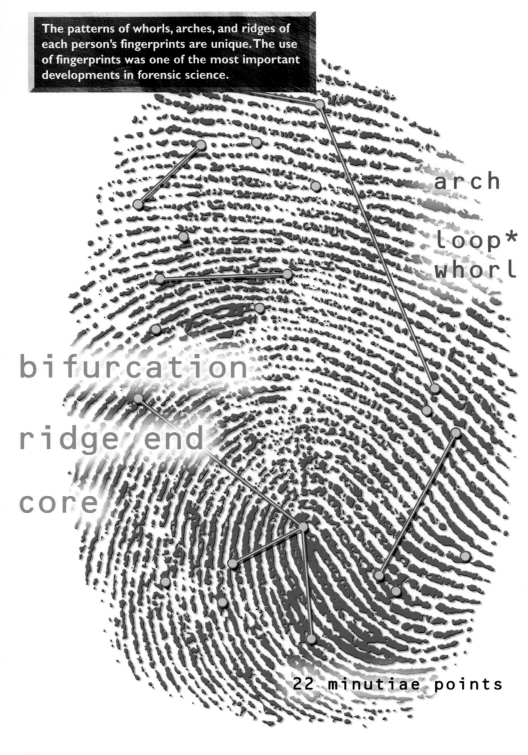

The patterns of whorls, arches, and ridges of each person's fingerprints are unique. The use of fingerprints was one of the most important developments in forensic science.

arch

loop*

whorl

bifurcation

ridge end

core

22 minutiae points

THE DISCOVERY OF FINGERPRINTS AS A UNIQUE IDENTIFIER

Although new inventions such as the compound microscope and the forensics laboratory were important, the use of fingerprints was probably the most vital development in the history of forensic science. The use of fingerprints was one of the most important developments in the evolution of forensic science. Fingerprints are made up of patterns of ridges on the tips of a person's fingers. These ridges can be made up of whorls, or circles; arches, or horizontal ridges; and loops, or backward-curving ridges. Every person's fingerprints are unique—no two people have the same set of fingerprints. Fingerprints have been used to identify people for thousands of years. In ancient times, people even signed contracts by marking their fingerprints with ink. The practice of using fingerprints to identify criminals, however, is less than two hundred years old.

During the mid-1800s, a Scottish doctor named Henry Faulds discovered that fingerprints grow back in the same pattern even if a person's skin is scraped or peeled off. Faulds spent many years working in Japan. One day, someone told him about a fingerprint that had been left by a thief on a dirty wall near Faulds's home. Faulds compared the print with one provided by a suspect and discovered they were different. The suspect was innocent. A few days later, another suspect was fingerprinted, and this time the prints matched. The second suspect was arrested for the crime.

When Faulds returned to England, he studied mummies in the British Museum and realized that fingerprints do not fade with age. He then wrote several letters to scientific journals in which he described his findings and called for a national registry of fingerprints. British police and officials, however, did not believe that anyone could be convicted based on fingerprint evidence, and Faulds was not taken seriously.

Meanwhile, other people were also discovering the importance of fingerprints. In 1858, William Herschel, an Englishman working for the British government in India, announced that no two people had the same fingerprints. His ideas were later developed by English scientist Sir Francis Galton.

Galton had studied Bertillonage, the system of identifying criminals by photographing and measuring them, and was very interested in identifying people based on body features. He analyzed fingerprints and announced that there should be twelve identical points on two sets of fingerprints in order to establish a match. Because Galton was well respected, his views were widely accepted.

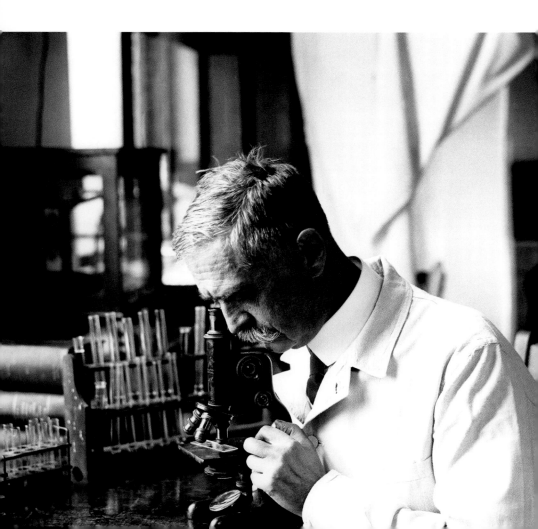

THE HENRY SYSTEM

Fingerprint identification continued to improve. During the late 1800s, Edward Henry of Scotland Yard developed a method to categorize fingerprints by their patterns of whorls, arches, and ridges. This system became known as the Henry System, and it is still used today.

By the early 1900s, fingerprints were being used by police departments around the world as a way to identify and capture criminals. At the time, fingerprints were analyzed simply by looking at them and comparing one set to another. If enough points matched, the fingerprints were considered to be from the same person and could be used as a positive identification.

BLOOD TYPES

Another part of the human body that has become an important tool in forensic science is blood. In the early 1900s, an Austrian doctor named Karl Landsteiner discovered that there were four different blood types, which he called types A, B, AB, and O. Different antigens, or chemical compounds, in the blood create the different blood types.

The discovery of different blood types allowed forensic scientists to tell whether the blood at a crime scene belonged to the victim or to someone else. Blood could also be matched to criminal suspects. Occasionally the blood at a crime scene might belong to an animal, but investigators could quickly determine this because animal blood and human blood contain different chemicals.

Dr. Karl Landsteiner's discovery that there are four different types of human blood gave investigators another way to identify suspects.

DETERMINING THE TIME OF DEATH

Even early investigators understood that in addition to establishing identity, it was important to determine exactly when a person died in order to solve a crime. The ancient Chinese book *The Washing Away of Wrongs* described how corpses decomposed at different rates of speed during different seasons of the year. For example, bodies decomposed more quickly during the hot summer months than they did during cold winter weather, because heat quickens the process of decomposition.

If a body was found shortly after death, ancient scientists noted three characteristics that could help determine when the person died: *rigor mortis*, *livor mortis*, and *algor mortis*. *Rigor mortis* is the stiffening of the body. Immediately after death, the body is limp and soft, but as the hours pass, the muscles tighten and the body becomes stiff and hard. After about thirty-six hours, however, the stiffness disappears.

Livor mortis, or lividity, refers to the discoloration that results from the settling of blood inside the body. For example, if a person dies while sitting down, the blood will settle in the lower parts of the body and turn these parts pink. As time passes, this color darkens to dark red, purple, and dark blue, and the discoloration remains even if the body is moved after death. Finally, *algor mortis* is the cooling of the body, which was probably one of the earliest observations people made about corpses. Bodies cool after death, and in general, the cooler the body, the longer it has been dead.

DECAY

Bodies that have been dead for more than a few days provide even more clues about the time of death. The first is putrefaction, or the decay caused by bacteria inside the body. Decay usually starts in the

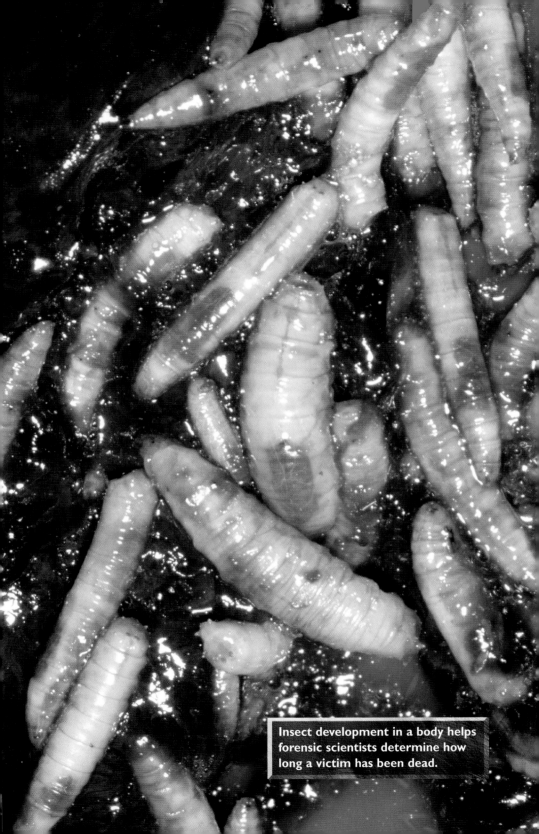

Insect development in a body helps forensic scientists determine how long a victim has been dead.

stomach, where there is a lot of naturally occurring bacteria, and then moves up into the chest and down the legs and arms. As the days pass, the decay spreads and changes the color and texture of the body. It also produces an unpleasant odor.

In time, the smell of the decaying body attracts insects. Scientists can study how long insects have been on a body by seeing if they have laid eggs that developed into adults. Based on the length of the life cycles of particular insects, forensic scientists can determine how long a body has been dead. For example, a body that contains several generations of insects has been dead a long time.

The history of the science of forensics, like that of most other scientific fields, has been a long, slow advance interrupted by important developments that greatly changed the field. The progress continues today. In recent years, new technologies such as computers and new techniques such as DNA testing have again transformed the practice of forensic science.

BERTILLONAGE

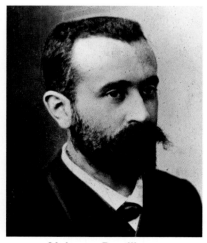

Alphonse Bertillon

In 1879, a man named Alphonse Bertillon was working as a clerk in the records office of Paris's Judicial Identification System. Bertillon believed that no two people had the same measurements. He developed a system of identifying criminals by photographing and measuring them that became known as Bertillonage.

Bertillonage became quite popular in France. When a suspect was arrested, the police took a

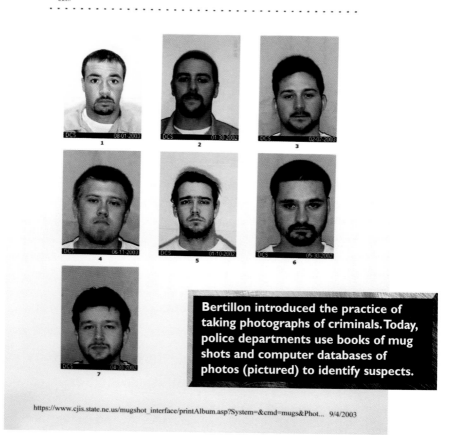

Bertillon introduced the practice of taking photographs of criminals. Today, police departments use books of mug shots and computer databases of photos (pictured) to identify suspects.

https://www.cjis.state.ne.us/mugshot_interface/printAlbum.asp?System=&cmd=mugs&Phot... 9/4/2003

series of body measurements, including the size of the head and the length of the feet. These measurements were recorded and could be used to identify criminals.

Bertillon also developed the practice of photographing criminals. Each suspect's face was photographed from the front and the side. These photographs were then put into a book, which could be given to victims to help them identify criminals. Although Bertillonage is not used anymore, police departments around the world still use books of photos, called mug shots, to identify criminals today.

THE PARKMAN CASE

In 1849, a medical professor named Dr. George Parkman went to see Dr. John White Webster at his laboratory at Harvard Medical School. Parkman wanted to get back some money that Webster owed him.

Parkman was never seen again. Although police searched Webster's laboratory and office, they could not find any evidence that Parkman had been there or that a crime had been committed. Webster claimed that he had paid Parkman and watched him leave the office.

A discovery by the school's janitor, however, showed that Webster's story was a lie. The janitor found body parts in part of the school where dead bodies were stored for use by medical students. After the janitor told police what he had found, they checked Webster's office again. This time, they found some bones in a chest and a set of false teeth in the furnace.

Several medical experts were brought in to study the bones and teeth. They decided that the bones were the right age and size to be Parkman's. Then Parkman's dentist mentioned that he had made a set of false teeth for Parkman a few years earlier. He produced a plaster cast he had created when he made the teeth, and the cast and the false teeth matched perfectly.

After he heard the evidence against him, Webster confessed that he had killed Parkman and cut up the body. He was convicted of murder and executed in 1850.

CHAPTER 2

FORENSICS TODAY

Forensic science in the twenty-first century has become highly sophisticated and extremely accurate. Although scientific techniques have changed dramatically over the past two hundred years, collecting and identifying fingerprints remains one of the most important methods of identifying criminals and solving crimes.

There are three different types of fingerprints: patent, impressed, and latent. Patent fingerprints are left when a person's hands are covered with a wet material such as grease, paint, or blood. Impressed fingerprints are left in a soft surface, such as candle wax or a piece of chocolate. Both patent and impressed fingerprints are fairly easy to spot.

The third type of fingerprints, latent prints, are the most common, but they are also the most difficult to find. Latent fingerprints are left by oils and sweat on the surface of the skin and are invisible to the naked eye. Investigators must use special tools to find them.

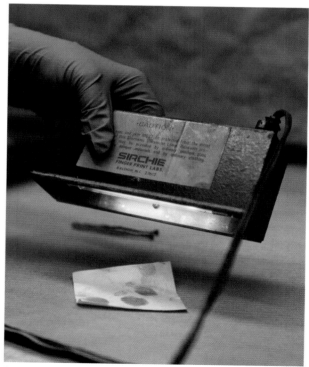

Investigators use special tools to find latent fingerprints, which are otherwise invisible.

TAKING PRINTS

To find and preserve latent fingerprints, investigators use brushes to dust an aluminum powder over the crime scene. The aluminum powder, which is used because it reflects light and is easy to see,

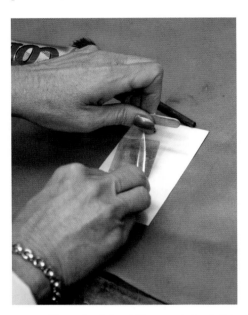

sticks to the moisture in the latent prints. The prints are then collected by using special tape to lift them from the surface. The dusting powder sticks to the tape and create a perfect picture of the fingerprint. The print is then taken to a crime laboratory to be studied, photographed, and cataloged.

Because fingerprints can be left on many different surfaces, scientists have developed

To make latent fingerprints visible, investigators can dust the prints with aluminum powder then lift them with special tape (above), or apply chemicals that glow (below).

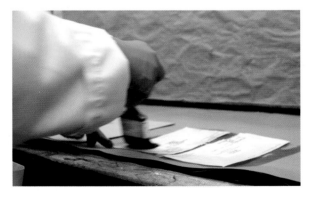

different dusting powders to suit particular circumstances. For example, heated iodine crystals work better than aluminum dust to capture fingerprints left on paper. Another chemical called DFO (diazafluorenone) reacts to acids in the fingerprints and glows to reveal the prints.

ANALYZING FINGERPRINTS

One hundred years ago, the only way to match sets of fingerprints was for a person to look at them and try to find similarities. Today, powerful computers are used to match similar features on sets of fingerprints. When a set of fingerprints is taken, it is entered into a computer database that can be quickly searched to see if any existing prints match the new set. Most countries today have national fingerprint databases that allow investigators to compare thousands of fingerprints per second and search a much larger collection than one person doing the job by sight alone.

THE FORENSIC USE OF DENTAL RECORDS

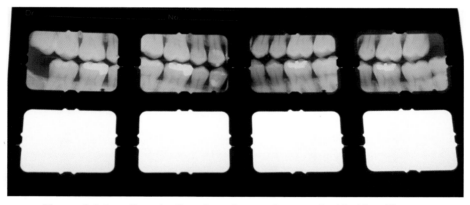

X rays (pictured) and other dental records are valuable identifiers of both suspects and victims.

Another unique part of a person's body is the teeth. Most adults have thirty-two teeth, although some may have been lost because of disease or injury. Teeth are difficult to destroy, so they provide valuable evidence of a person's identity after death. Investigators can check dental records to find out if a person is missing teeth, how many fillings he or she has, and other identifying details. Since no two people have the exact same dental histories, dental identification is highly accurate and can provide an important clue to solve a mysterious death. The use of X rays in modern dentistry has greatly helped forensic scientists, because they can not only read a dentist's records about a particular patient, but see pictures of the victim's teeth as well.

Dental records can also be used to find an attacker or murderer. Sometimes attackers bite their victim and leave a telltale impression on the body. Scientists can photograph and measure the bite and compare it to dental records to identify the attacker. Details such as how far apart the teeth are or the shape and size of the mouth also provide a unique identifying tool.

THE FORENSIC USE OF HAIR SAMPLES

Body hair can also provide important clues about how a person died. When a body is discovered under mysterious circumstances, investigators take hair samples to analyze in a laboratory. Hair samples are not just taken from the head, but from other parts of

Analysis of hair samples can reveal clues to a victim's identity and how he or she died.

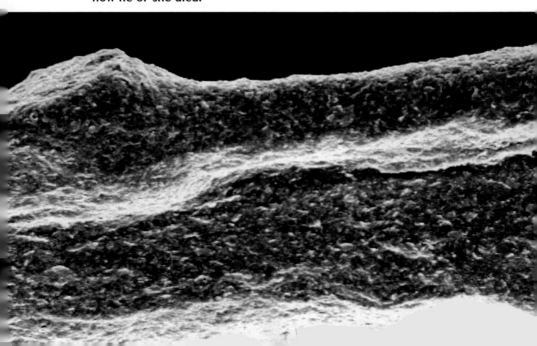

the body, too, because drugs or poisons can show up in different concentrations in different parts of the body. So while a hair taken from a victim's head may not show a certain poison, hair taken from another part of the same body might reveal the chemical.

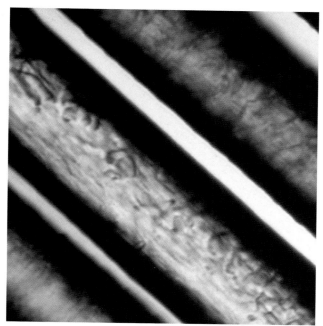

Forensic scientists treat hair samples with chemical solutions that react with poisons, chemicals, and drugs.

When a hair sample is brought to the laboratory, it is washed to remove any shampoos, cosmetics, or other foreign materials and cut into half-inch lengths. Each specimen is then treated with several different chemical solutions that react with poisons, chemicals, and drugs such as heroin, cocaine, and marijuana. If chemicals are found in a person's hair, investigators can even pinpoint when they were ingested. Since everyone's hair grows about half an inch every month, investigators can tell almost precisely when a chemical entered the body by its location on the hair shaft.

Hair can also help investigators identify victims by providing important clues to his or her identity. For example, different races have different types of hair. A black person's hair tends to be curly and coarse, while an Asian person usually has straight, fine hair. Each strand of hair has three layers: the medulla, which is the innermost core of the hair; the cortex, which contains the hair's color; and the cuticle, or outer covering. A white person's hair has more evenly distributed bits of pigment in the cortex than a black person's hair. Asian hair has a long, straight medulla, while other races have fragmented medullas. All of these differences can help forensic investigators to identify a victim or a criminal.

DNA TESTING

The use of deoxyribonucleic acid (DNA) testing is probably the most important development in forensic science since the widespread use of fingerprinting. DNA is found in the nucleus of every cell in the body except red blood cells, which do not have a nucleus. It is made up of a chain of four chemicals: adenine, guanine, cytosine, and thymine. These chemicals can combine in an infinite number of ways, which means that no two people—except identical twins—have the same DNA.

There are two kinds of DNA: mitochondrial DNA and nuclear DNA. Mitochondrial DNA is inherited only from a person's mother and is most easily extracted in hair strands and bones. Since siblings have the same mitochondrial DNA, it is not the most useful type of DNA to use for identification purposes.

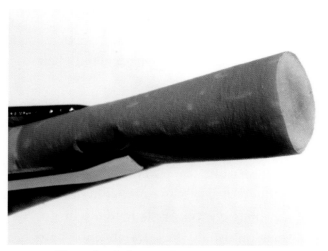

The saliva left on a cigarette butt provides DNA evidence that forensic scientists can use to identify suspects and victims.

Nuclear DNA, however, contains one strand of DNA from a person's mother and one strand from the father. Nuclear DNA is unique to each person and is easily extracted from the cells inside the mouth and the roots of the hair. Saliva is an excellent source of nuclear DNA.

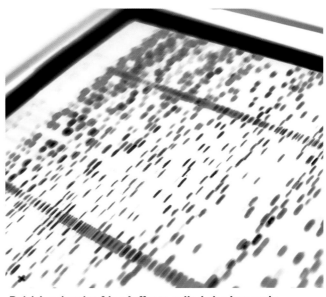

British scientist Alec Jeffreys called the bar-code pattern of a DNA sample (pictured) a DNA fingerprint because each band provides such specific information.

For many years, DNA was used only to identify genetic disorders and predict the chance of a person inheriting a tendency to develop certain diseases or conditions. Then, during the 1970s, a British scientist named Alec Jeffreys began to treat DNA with enzymes that caused a chemical reaction and broke the DNA into fragments.

On September 15, 1984, Jeffreys was looking at X rays of some specially treated DNA when he noticed that the samples appeared as a series of gray and black bands that looked like the bar codes on products in a supermarket. Jeffreys and the other scientists on his team realized they had made a great discovery—every series of bands was different because each DNA molecule held a specific pattern of information. Jeffreys called his discovery DNA fingerprinting. Like fingerprinting, DNA could be used to identify criminals and victims and solve crimes. Today, DNA testing has become an essential tool for modern forensic scientists.

A MODERN AUTOPSY

While fingerprints, hair samples, dental records, and DNA testing can help determine the identity of a criminal or victim, frequently the only way to determine the cause of death is to perform an autopsy. An autopsy is a thorough internal and external examination of a corpse that is usually performed by a specially trained doctor called a medical examiner.

Autopsies can provide many clues about the cause and circumstances of a person's death. The condition of the body can help the examiner decide when the person died, which helps

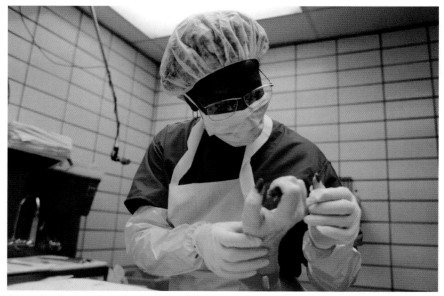

A medical examiner looks for evidence underneath a victim's fingernails and matches bloodstains on clothing to the victim's wounds.

investigators determine when a crime was committed and where possible suspects were at that time. Autopsies also reveal the cause of death through physical clues such as broken bones, gunshot wounds, or brain damage. Autopsies can also reveal that a person died from natural causes if the heart, liver, lungs, brain, or other major organs show signs of disease.

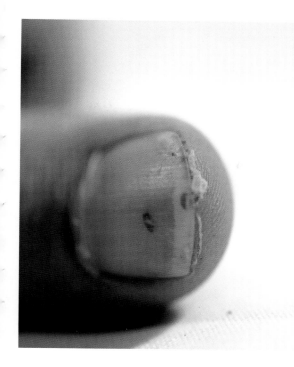

After the initial on-site investigation is completed, the medical examiner's office brings the body to the morgue in a body bag. Once at the morgue, the bag is placed on an examining table and the body is removed, weighed, measured, and photographed. The medical examiner inspects the outside of the body and records any signs of injury, such as bruises, cuts, or gunshot wounds. Any material found underneath the fingernails is removed and stored in a plastic bag.

Next, all clothes and jewelry are removed and stored for return to the victim's family or use as evidence in a trial. Blood or other stains on clothing will be matched to injuries on the body to help examiners determine what was happening when the victim was killed. If a person was shot or stabbed, for example,

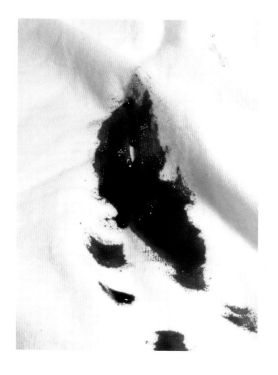

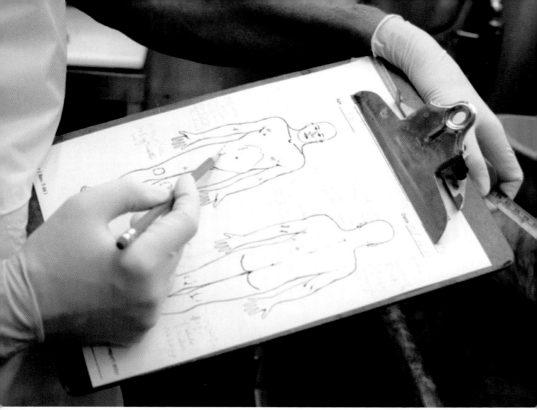

Before the autopsy begins, the medical examiner inspects the outside of a victim's body and notes any signs of injury.

the position of a bloodstain on a shirt can indicate which direction the weapon came from. Powder marks from a gun on clothing or skin can establish that a victim was shot at very close range.

Once the external inspection is complete, the internal examination begins. Using a scalpel, the medical examiner makes a Y-shaped cut from the left shoulder to the right shoulder, and then down the chest and stomach. The skin is pulled back to reveal the organs inside.

The medical examiner removes each organ and examines it for possible clues. For example, if a person has died from carbon monoxide poisoning, his or her muscles will be bright pink. If the sac around the heart is filled with blood, the victim probably received a violent blow to the chest. Examiners take samples of damaged organs or tissues for later use as evidence in a trial.

In addition to looking at each organ, the medical examiner also takes samples of all bodily fluids, including blood and urine. The contents of the victim's stomach are also removed and analyzed. Toxicologists can examine these fluids and discover the presence of many foreign substances, such as drugs, alcohol, or poison.

After examining the torso, the medical examiner cuts open the skull with a special saw and removes the brain. The brain is carefully checked for bruises, blood clots, or swelling that might indicate a blow to the head.

Once all the organs have been examined, they are placed back inside the body. The incisions are sewn closed and the body is released to a funeral home for burial preparations. Autopsies usually take several hours, although the length depends on the condition of the body and the circumstances of the death.

Toxicologists test blood and other bodily fluids for the presence of foreign substances.

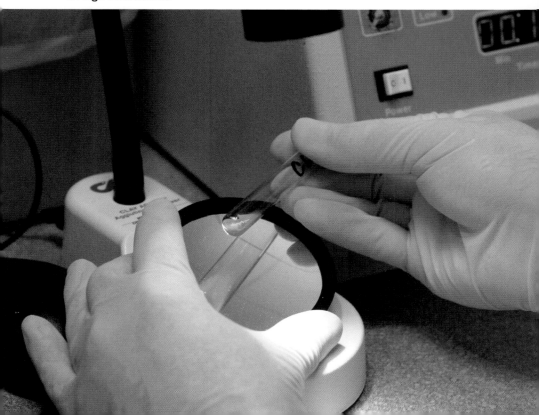

CLUES FROM THE CRIME SCENE

The body is not the only place where clues are found. Frequently the place where the victim was found is a treasure trove of information. The area around the body is searched for tiny clues, such as carpet fibers or tiny fragments of soil or plant material. Every bit of evidence is picked up, either with tweezers or by scraping or swabbing the surface, and placed in a plastic bag. Later, investigators will look at each piece of evidence under a compound microscope.

Bloodstains and trace materials like carpet fibers from a crime scene can provide important clues to a suspect's identity.

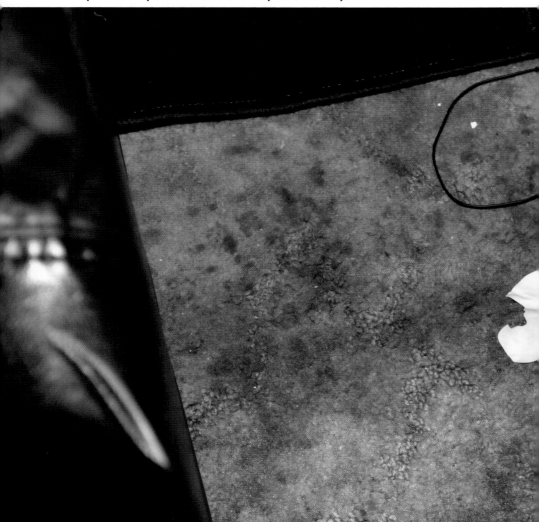

TRACE MATERIALS

The scene of a crime is often loaded with clues in the form of trace materials, such as fibers from the killer's clothes, and are sometimes found on the victim. Such evidence can prove a connection between killer and victim. Similarly, if carpet fibers found on the body match those in a suspect's house, this establishes a physical link between the suspect and the victim.

Trace materials can also indicate if a body was moved after death. For example, if a body is found on a paved surface but has bits of plants or soil on it, it is likely that the body was moved from somewhere else. Similarly, if a body is found outside but has carpet fibers on it, the body was probably moved from an indoor location.

BLOODSTAINS

Blood spatters at the scene also provide important clues. The shape and size of a drop of blood can tell a trained scientist how far the drop fell and from which direction. These clues can help investigators re-create the crime scene and figure out where the victim was when he or she was attacked.

Today, even hidden blood can be examined. After a violent crime or accident, blood often spatters all over the area and leaves tiny specks of blood that are difficult to find. Investigators use a chemical called luminol to find hidden blood. Luminol is applied to surfaces at the scene, and if it comes into contact with blood, it glows, leading investigators to even the tiniest drop of blood.

From the time of Julius Caesar to today, forensics has evolved into an important and complicated science. Modern techniques of forensic science, including computerized analysis of fingerprints and DNA testing, represent great advances in the ability of science to help the law. In the future, there are certainly more surprises in store.

NOT JUST FINGERS

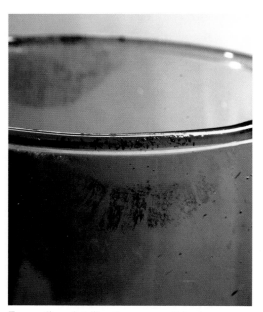

Even a lip print like the one on this glass can help investigators identify a criminal or victim.

Fingers are not the only part of the body that leave prints. The same oils that are found on a person's fingers are also found on a person's feet, the palms of the hands, the ears, and the lips. These parts of the body also have wrinkles, lines, and other features that create a unique pattern. Investigators can dust and preserve prints from these body parts as well and use them to identify criminals and bodies.

RECONSTRUCTING HEADS

Sometimes bodies are found, but no one can figure out who they are because the face or skull have decomposed or been badly damaged. In these cases, specialists can reconstruct, or rebuild, the skull and face to create an image of the person's appearance. Facial reconstruction begins with a cast of the skull. Plastic balls are used for eyes, and the flesh is re-created in clay. Facial features can be determined by the shape of the skull and the position of the bones. The whole process can be done in about a day.

Once the reconstruction is complete, the figure can be photographed and shown in newspapers, on television, and over the Internet. As a result, someone may recognize the figure and be able to identify the body.

FINDING THE GUILTY—AND THE INNOCENT

DNA testing has been used as evidence in many criminal trials, and it has sent many people to prison for their crimes. DNA testing has also, however, been used to free people who were wrongly convicted and sent to prison for crimes they did not commit.

One of the most high-profile cases involving DNA evidence was known as the Central Park jogger case. On April 19, 1989, a woman was raped, beaten, and left for dead while she was jogging in New

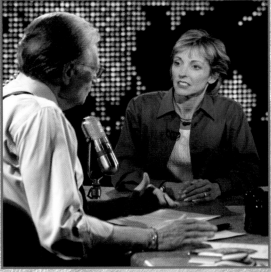

DNA evidence in the case of the Central Park jogger, pictured here as a guest on *Larry King Live*, proved that the boys convicted of the crime were innocent.

York City's Central Park. Five teenage boys were soon arrested and confessed to the crime. They were convicted and sentenced to seven to thirteen years in prison, even though no physical evidence tied them to the victim.

Thirteen years later, a convicted rapist named Matias Reyes admitted that he had attacked and raped the Central Park jogger. A DNA test of semen found on the victim's body confirmed Reyes's story. The five men originally convicted of the crime had their sentences overturned, but by then they had already served many years in jail.

CHAPTER 3

THE FUTURE OF FORENSICS

Computers have changed the world of forensic science and made it much easier to analyze data. In the past, all forensic analysis had to be done by hand. For example, fingerprints were matched by a person who looked at different sets of prints. This method of visual identification took a long time and limited the number of prints one person could look at. It also created the risk that the person could make a mistake and either miss or overlook a match.

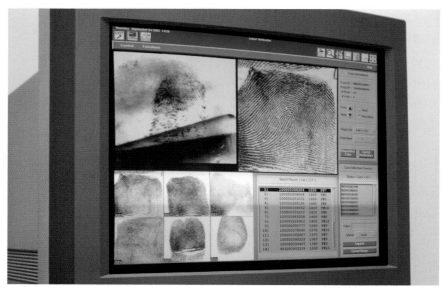

Computers enable investigators to quickly compare a fingerprint to hundreds of thousands of other fingerprints in a national database.

Computers have made it easy to compare vast sets of data. Investigators can not only match hundreds of thousands of fingerprints from a national database, they can also match other evidence. A serial murderer may kill his or her victims the same way, leave the body in the same position, or leave a specific piece of physical evidence at the scene of each crime. Computer programs can analyze these details and come up with matches that allow investigators to see patterns in crimes.

Computers can also analyze data from accidents. Perhaps victims of car crashes are injured in the same way because of a

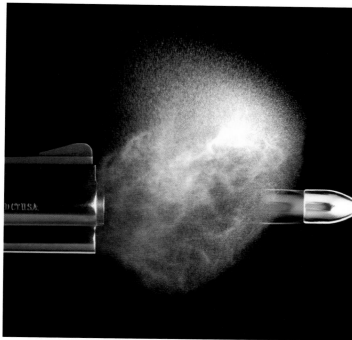

Computer-aided ballistics analyzes the path of a bullet once it leaves a gun.

fault in the car's construction. Identifying such a fault can show carmakers how to redesign the car so it is safer. Data from accident scenes can identify dangerous intersections and suggest ways to make them safer, such as adding a traffic light or improving sight lines.

Computer scientists are always creating new computer models. Some computer programs study ballistics, or the science of an object's motion in flight. Ballistics usually focuses on what happens when a bullet is fired from a gun. One recent computer model analyzes the path a bullet travels and how the blood spatters from the wound. This data can show what position the shooter was in when he or she fired the gun and help investigators re-create a murder scene. This type of analysis used to be done by a forensic artist who made measurements and sketched possible outcomes by hand. A computer can do the work more quickly and efficiently and print out results that are easier to understand.

FORENSIC MAPPING

Computers can also help forensic scientists obtain more accurate measurements at a crime scene. For example, investigators will measure how far the body is from other objects in the area. If bullets are found on the floor or in the walls, their distance from the body is also measured. These measurements tell the story of the crime. When they are taken by hand, however, as they used to be, the process could take a long time and was not always accurate.

Today, a new technology called forensic mapping is changing how measurements are taken. Forensic mapping measures different angles to document physical evidence.

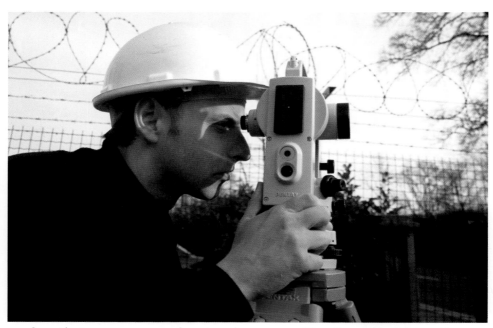

Investigators measure angles at a crime scene with a theodolite (pictured) to create a forensic map of the area.

To create a forensic map, an investigator places a special box called a total station at the crime scene. The total station includes four parts. The theodolite is a device that measures angles. The electronic distance measuring instrument, or EDMI, uses infrared light to measure distances. A prism reflects the infrared light so it can be measured by the theodolite. Finally, a data collector captures the measurements and records them.

The investigator sets up the total station at several points at the scene in order to measure all relevant distances and angles. After the measurements are collected and stored in a data collector, they are brought to the lab and downloaded to a mapping software program. This computer program uses geometric measurements to read the locations and assign a code number to each one. Finally, the software uses these codes to display an accurate map of the scene.

Forensic mapping can be used on horizontal surfaces, such as the floor or the ground. It is also useful for measuring vertical surfaces. Sometimes, investigators will find blood spatters or bullet marks on a vertical surface, such as a wall or a door. Forensic mapping can measure the distances between these clues and the body, which gives investigators more information to work with.

ADVANCES IN DNA TESTING

DNA testing is constantly changing and improving. Scientists are creating new technologies that will allow them to match DNA using much smaller samples than is possible today. One method is to treat the DNA with different chemicals in order to identify different markers to make matches. The more markers that can be used in a sample, the better the odds of identifying that sample and possibly matching it to a victim or killer to solve a mysterious death. Using more markers will also make DNA testing more accurate.

In addition, scientists are also working to identify degraded DNA, which is DNA taken from bodies that have already decomposed or been severely damaged. One laboratory studies the sequence of chemicals in a strand of DNA. They have been able to identify samples that contained just seventy-two chemicals on one strand. This number is likely to get smaller as technology improves. In time, DNA that is too small or not suitable to make matches today will be good enough to make matches in the future. DNA molecules can survive for a long time, which means that samples of bone, body tissue, or blood from old crime scenes can be tested years later, when new techniques are developed or new evidence is collected.

Another goal is to make DNA testing more efficient and cost-effective. Science has already made great advances in this area. Procedures that used to take months and cost tens of thousands of dollars can now be performed in days for as little as $250 per test. An instrument called an automated mass spectrometer performed up to one hundred DNA analyses in just one hour in a recent test. This procedure is likely to be available to commercial testing laboratories in the next few years.

Soon, DNA evidence may be able to be analyzed right at the crime scene by using a portable DNA-testing machine. Although testing at the scene probably would not be as thorough as laboratory testing, it could be used to check DNA samples and help investigators focus their attention on the most likely suspects during the crucial hours immediately after a crime has been committed.

Many states have begun to put together DNA databases. These states require all convicted criminals to provide a DNA sample. These samples are stored on a computer and can be quickly matched to DNA evidence taken from crime scenes. For this system to work properly, DNA evidence from all crime scenes must also be collected and stored, so that both pieces of the puzzle are available to match up. These matches can solve crimes that occurred years ago. In time, it is likely that the United States will have a national database for DNA, just as it does for fingerprints. Other countries, such as the United Kingdom and Canada, have already created national DNA databases.

Advances in DNA technology will allow investigators to match very small samples of DNA (pictured) to criminals and victims.

CLINICAL FORENSIC PATHOLOGY

A DNA database uses material from live humans to solve crimes. Another way forensic scientists study the living is through forensic pathology. This relatively new science pathology sends forensics experts into hospital emergency rooms all over the country. These

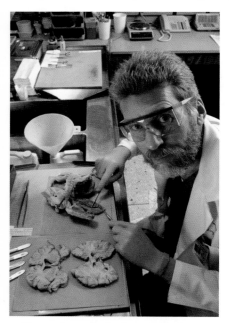

Forensic pathologists study how different types of physical trauma affect the human body.

experts are there to study injuries suffered by victims of violent crimes or accidents. Comparing their injuries to the ones on dead bodies helps pathologists gather more information about how various traumas affect body systems. This leads to more accurate determinations at crime scenes and helps investigators figure out how and why a person died—and who might have killed him or her. It can also help scientists when they conduct autopsies by providing them with the knowledge of how the human body is affected by trauma.

A CHANGING SCIENCE

Forensics is constantly changing and improving. From the discovery of what killed Julius Caesar more than two thousand years ago to today's high-tech crime labs, every piece of evidence is analyzed and fit into the puzzle of an unsolved crime. Each new development in forensics makes it easier to solve the puzzles that surround many deaths. These developments can even reach back into the past and help us solve crimes and other mysteries that happened decades or even centuries ago.

Of course, crimes still remain unsolved. With every advance in forensic science, though, it becomes more and more likely that one day there will be no such thing as a perfect crime. Meanwhile, forensic scientists, pathologists, police investigators, and laboratory technicians continue their work, uncovering the secrets of death and finding more and more pieces to solve crime-scene mysteries.

DNA AND THE WORLD TRADE CENTER

The attack on the World Trade Center was a landmark case in terms of DNA identification of a large number of victims. The sudden death of nearly three thousand people presented a challenge for forensic scientists like no other. Although some intact bodies were

Scientists hope that advances in DNA testing will allow them to identify many more of the victims of the September 11, 2001, attack on the World Trade Center.

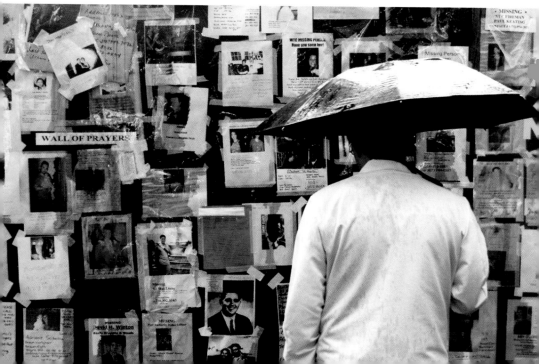

recovered, many were destroyed by the fire and the collapse of the buildings. Many of the remains were just body parts or fragments of bones or teeth. In addition, many of these body parts had been damaged by fire, heat, or water at the scene.

Another problem was obtaining a computer system to match more than twenty thousand remains with hair and saliva samples provided by the victims' families. Several corporations were given the job of creating computer programs to tackle the vast number of matches. Several laboratories also went to work and invented new ways to identify people based on small or damaged samples of DNA.

Two years after the disaster, slightly more than half of the victims had been positively identified. Scientists have not stopped working on the problem, however. Human remains that have not been identified yet are stored for the future. As scientists come up with new techniques to identify DNA using smaller and smaller samples, it is likely that many more victims of this disaster will be identified.

GLOSSARY

autopsy an examination of a body to determine the cause of death.

coroner an official who investigates unnatural deaths.

decompose to rot or decay.

enzymes proteins that cause chemical reactions to occur.

evidence information that proves something.

fibers tiny threads.

fragment a tiny piece.

morgue a place where dead bodies are kept until the family identifies and claims them.

pathology the study of diseases and their effect on the body.

toxicologist a person who studies poisons and their effect on the body.

FOR FURTHER INFORMATION

Books

Campbell, Andrea, *Forensic Science: Evidence, Clues, and Investigation.* Philadelphia: Chelsea House, 2000.

Fridell, Ron, *Solving Crimes: Pioneers of Forensic Science.* New York: Franklin Watts, 2000.

Jones, Charlotte Foltz, *Fingerprints and Talking Bones: How Real-Life Crimes Are Solved.* New York: Delacorte Press, 1997.

Lane, Brian, *Crime and Detection.* New York: Knopf, 1998.

Yeatts, Tabatha, *Forensics: Solving the Crime.* Minneapolis, MN: Oliver Press, 2001.

Websites

Crime Scene Investigations
www.crime-scene-investigator.net
Features guidelines for evidence collection, articles, and helpful resources and links.

Forensic Education and Consulting
http://forensicdna.com
Features a timeline of the history of forensics, a bibliography, and information about careers in the field.

Zeno's Forensic Site
http://forensic.to/forensic.html
An extensive list of resources and links on a variety of forensic science topics.

ABOUT THE AUTHOR

Joanne Mattern is the author of more than one hundred nonfiction and fiction books for children. Her favorite subjects are animals and nature, but she has also written biographies of explorers and sports figures, an encyclopedia on American immigration, classic novel retellings, and activity books. Ms. Mattern lives in New York State with her husband and young daughters.

INDEX